First published by Spank The Tomato LLC 2025

Copyright © 2025 by K. Savelesky

All rights reserved. No part of this publication may be reproduced, stored or transmitted in any form or by any means, electronic, mechanical, photocopying, recording, scanning, or otherwise without written permission from the publisher. It is illegal to copy this book, post it to a website, or distribute it by any other means without permission. K. Savelesky asserts the moral right to be identified as the author of this work. K. Savelesky has no responsibility for the persistence or accuracy of URLsfor external or third-party Internet Websites referred to in this publication and does not guarantee that any content on such Websites is, or will remain, accurate or appropriate. Designations used by companies to distinguish their products are often claimed as trademarks. All brand names and product names used in this book and on its cover are trade names, service marks, trademarks and registered trademarks of their respective owners. The publishers and the book are not associated with any product or vendor mentioned in this book. None of the companies referenced within the book have endorsed the book. It is up to the reader to research and verify information provided in this book. The author takes no responsibility for interpretation of information provided or claims made.

First edition

To my wonderful husband

For his never ending support and love.

May the adventures continue for another 30 years!

Table of Conents

Publication Protections

Prologue

Chapter 1 The Lowdown

Chapter 2 Why Try?

Chapter 3 Baby Steps

Chapter 4 Write it Down

Chapter 5 Check List

To those I've never met, but owe so much!

About the Author

Reviews and Contact

Prologue

For hundreds of years our ancestor's population didn't have cancer, obesity and autoimmune problems at alarming levels. They had other problems. While we have managed to overcome many of their problems, we have created new ones.

Now, in a world where it seems hard to escape from plastics and chemicals, I show you easy ways to mitigate the exposure. Our bodies aren't built to deal with the chemical intense environment that most of us live in. If (like me) you have been looking for easy ways to limit your exposure, have an impact on your health and well being then you've grabbed the right book!

I have kept this short and sweet on purpose, while trying not to sacrifice comprehensive research. There is so much more out there, but (like you) I am pretty busy with life. So! Here's the important stuff. I hope it helps you on your journey to a healthier home.

The Lowdown

You know systems have deteriorated for you when you (as a whole) have started to deteriorate. Approximately 18 years into our now 30-year marriage we began to take our life, habits and goals more seriously. We had never really been big on eating out, so that was one bad habit that was easy to ditch. We grew so serious about our own food prep that we started a YouTube instructional channel in 2018. Our local farmer became a favorite outing and we learned how to can our own tomatoes. I purchased organic cotton grocery bags (that we still have today) and made an effort to keep them in the car so I would never forget them. We got our blood vitamin levels tested and started taking targeted vitamins (not multi). It was a start. **Sometimes you just need a few simple beginnings to start seeing the bigger picture**.

In 2020 We packed up left our home of 25 years in Walla Walla, Washington to move to Newcastle, Wyoming. What I loved immediately were the people, the toughness of life and the beauty of the sky without pollution. It's a great place for someone interested in preparedness to really dig in and start learning, start doing and feel the meaning of life in your core being. Gratitude became my mantra. This phase of life began for us just before the supply shortages became a reality world wide. I started with rice, beans and the 5 gallons of canned tomatoes I had processed right before the move. I watched hours of videos and discovered places on line for my non consumables, vacuum sealer and dried goods (pastas) that were not available here. Living in a town of 3500 people with the nearest big shopping 1.5 hours away teaches resourcefulness. Organic groceries are not "a thing" and most folks don't care about it. The folks that know better go to the farmers market and local farmer for everything they need. Sustenance is very seasonal. We had a thing or 5 to learn. If I'm breaking the learning curves down by years, it looks something like this:

Year 1. Get our bearings and deal with the "new norm" of COVID (which was mostly ignored here). Expand our knowledge of electrical, plumbing and how to bail out a basement. Learn how to live without a fully functional heating system when its -20 out. Source firewood, eggs, milk, meat and labor (to help with renovating our new home). Mark settles into his first job. Watch tons of videos on prepping and health.

Year 2. Work on the house. Find a hormone specialist (took 5 tries and the keeper is in Colorado). Make connections with local farmers. Can more tomatoes. Add to our food stores a little bit every month. Start a home renovation business. End the home renovation business. Watch tons of videos on health. Change up our vitamins. Try carnivore.

Year 3 & 4. Quit smoking. Work on the house. Fix problems that other local contractors created. We tried our hand at road construction traffic control. Mark starts working for the coal mining company. I continue with renovations on our home. Watch tons of videos on health. Change up our vitamins. Quit drinking alcohol. I have precancerous polyps removed from my colon. Mark gets diagnosed with prostate cancer. Watch tons of videos on health and replacing plastic in our life. Reduce our vitamins. 3 months carnivore. **Now** it's time to get serious….

Why Try?

Science on plastics and forever chemicals found in body tissues and even brain tissue is coming to our attention. Research is increasing and the data is alarming. I will share some of my resources in this book, but a basic Brave browser search with AI is how I find a lot of my information. I highly encourage you to ultimately…Do your own research.

This is located in pub med: https://pmc.ncbi.nlm.nih.gov/articles/PMC11342020/

Summary of presence of microplastics in human body systems including their characteristics and possible pathway of microplastics into the body. Schematic representations were generated by BioRender.com. ABS – Acrylonitrile Butadiene Styrene, CA – Cellulose Acetate, CPE – Chlorinated Polyethylene, EPS – Expanded Polystyrene, mm – millimetre, PA – Polyamide, PAN – Polyacrylonitrile, PBS – Phosphate-buffered Saline, PES – Polyethersulfone, PE – Polyethylene, PET – Polyethylene Terephthalate, PC – Polycarbonate, PMMA – Polymethyl Methacrylate, POM – Polyoxymethylene, PP – Polypropylene, PS – Polystyrene, PSF/PSU – Polysulfone, PU/PUR – Polyurethane, PTFE – Polytetrafluoroethylene, PVC –

Polyvinyl Chloride, TPE – Thermoplastic Elastomers, SEBS – Styrene-Ethylene-Butylene-Styrene, µm – micrometre.

I worry for babies and little kids the most. Their small bodies aren't designed to deal with these types of overloads. It's being argued that plastics and chemicals are a big contributor to childhood illnesses.

Dr. Rhonda Patrick is a scientist we both follow on YouTube. She has podcasts that go rather extensively into micro plastics and the chemicals in plastics (even "food safe"). Another pod caster, Dr. Paul Saladino has lots of good information as well and is fun to watch.

Plastic isn't the only thing poisoning us. Highly processed foods contain toxins that aren't even required to be listed on the package. *Generally Recognized as Safe* is often seen on labeling. Just think about that for a minute. I'd personally prefer "Absolutely 100% Good for You", but I don't have a say in the FDA. As I am preparing to publish this, the government is making much needed changes to food ingredient standards and banning several harmful products.

I am wary of anything that I can smell. If you can smell it then you are breathing it. I ***used* to be** a big fan of scented candles, perfumes and products that cover bad odors. Skin care products are things to be extra aware of. Your skin absorbs these things into your body.

I'm a believer in the receipt conspiracy. I got this from an AI Brave search. **Receipts can be harmful to touch due to the presence of toxic chemicals like bisphenol S (BPS) and bisphenol A (BPA) on thermal paper**. These chemicals can be absorbed through the skin and have been linked to health issues such as hormone disruption, cognitive damage, decreased sperm count, and breast cancer. A recent study (678) found that holding a receipt for just 10 seconds can cause the skin to absorb enough BPS to exceed California's safety threshold. This is particularly concerning for cashiers and other retail workers who handle many receipts throughout the day.

Again…Do your own research.

Coated cookware can be problematic. Even if the coating is safe, what about the glue that gets exposed if you scratch it?

Lastly, I want to share what AI told me about microwave ovens and cell phones.

Research on the harms of microwave ovens has been extensive and it is largely concluded that they are safe when used correctly. However, there are some concerns and potential risks associated with their use:

1. **Radiation Leaks**: While microwave ovens are designed to contain radiation, there is a small risk of radiation leaks if the oven is damaged or improperly maintained. The U.S. Food and Drug Administration (FDA) sets strict standards to limit radiation leakage, but any damage to the oven, such as broken door hinges, latches, or seals, could increase the risk of leaks.
2. **Nutrient Loss**: Some studies suggest that microwaving can cause a loss of certain nutrients in food, particularly vitamin C and other heat-sensitive nutrients. However, microwave cooking can also preserve nutrients better than other cooking methods because it typically requires shorter cooking times.
3. **Plastic Containers**: There are concerns about the use of plastic containers in microwave ovens, as some plastics can release harmful chemicals when heated. This can potentially contaminate food and pose health risks.
4. **Uneven Heating**: Microwaves can heat food unevenly, which might lead to under cooked spots where bacteria can survive. This can increase the risk of food borne illnesses if food is not heated thoroughly.

5. **Superheating**: Another potential risk is superheating, where water or liquids can become heated beyond their boiling point without visible signs of boiling. This can lead to sudden boiling or splashing when the container is moved, causing burns.

Research on the harms of cell phones

Research on the harms of cell phones indicates that excessive use can lead to various health issues. One study found that problematic cell phone use can result in social and family conflicts, loss of interest in other activities, insomnia and sleep disturbance. Additionally, cell phone addiction can cause personal and social relationship problems, while putting jobs or studies in danger of being lost. Addiction to scrolling and reaction (positive and negative) can cause continued use despite awareness of negative effects.

Cell phones emit low levels of non-ionizing radiation, also known as radio frequency (RF) energy. While there is currently no consistent evidence that non-ionizing radiation increases cancer risk in humans, scientists are investigating a possible link between cell phone use and certain types of tumors, such as accoustic neuroma and glioma.

We haven't had a microwave for a couple of decades now. We would probably still be using it if we had it (convenience). We always use the speaker phone when talking on the cell phone. Cell phones are never worn on our person. The best way ***to be sure*** about either of these don't have a negative effect on you is to either not use them or limit usage as much as possible. I'm not even remotely interested in testing the toxic effect of anything listed above on myself.

Does the world feel totally hostile to you yet? I have some good news. There is hope and a path out of the toxic soup we call our environment. Mitigation and elimination are within reach.

Baby Steps

The easiest things to fix you can start doing right away. Stop using harmful products. Stop buying them. Stop replacing them with more junk. At minimum you should replace a product with non toxic alternative when your current supply runs out. I know it's hard to throw out a brand new bottle of dish soap or new sponges and if you can't bring yourself to do it….Don't replace it with more junk. Seed and vegetable oils should be thrown out FULL STOP!

The following is what I started halfheartedly years ago. This year I dug in, began pitching the bad and replacing it with the best that I can find and afford. It's understandable that the process can seem overwhelming at first, but it doesn't have to feel that way. Pick one thing, one area or one category and start chipping away as you can to replace the toxic things in your life. Several of these things will actually save you a lot of money.

Easiest things to do: Use Organic cotton grocery bags. Throw away plastics that touch your food. Don't buy food products in plastic. I do not put produce in the bags they provide. It sits nice and pretty in my cart, like it just came from the farm. Use baking soda and vinegar instead of cleaning chemicals. Use *old* olive oil as wood furniture polish. Use wash rags or coconut fiber pads instead of sponges. Stay out of the middle isles of the grocery store. Stick to the perimeter where the fresh whole foods are.

READ LABELS. If you can't pronounce it and are too lazy to look it up (like me most of the time), skip it.

Cheapest things to replace:

Utensils. Ice cube trays. Plastic containers. Tooth brushes. Floss. Drinking straws (ours are stainless steel and might not be suitable for kids). Toilet paper.

Investments to consider:

1. Ditch your microwave for a toaster oven.

2. Purchase a RFID Blocking cover for your cell phone from a reputable source.

3. Replace plastic kitchen machines with glass, stainless steel or cast iron (NOT COATED)

4. Reverse Osmosis water filter. I will eventually get a whole house one.

5. Air purifier

6. Bed and bedding. No VOC (volatile organic chemicals) furniture is best. 100% Organic Cotton bedding is ideal (also not as suseptable to static).

7. Recreational kitchen equipment such as ice cream makers and soda machines. (As far as I know, all cans are lined with plastic, even soda water).

Second hand stores and yard sales are great places to find a lot of kitchen supply replacements. We use dozens of quart canning jars to store leftovers in the fridge and dry goods on the shelves. It's nice to be able to see what is in the container before it becomes a Frankenstein science project. You can even freeze food and liquids in mason jars if you don't fill them all the way so there is room for expansion during the freezing process. An electric mason jar sealer can keep dry goods shelf stable for longer and while the only one I have found is plastic…It doesn't touch food and I will replace it with stainless steel the day one is made.

In a nutshell, I have decided that if I can:

1. Smell it and it's synthetic
2. Taste it and it's highly processed
3. Touch it to my skin and it's not recognizable by nature

It has to go or become extremely limited in my environment and treated with care.

If I don't know then the same rules apply. Technology can be a wonderful thing! I love that I can type this on a computer that will help me correct obvious errors. I love that I don't have to use white out paint to errase mistakes. I remember those days (yup! I'm that old). I love that I can send pics and messages instantly to friends and family.

I wish it were all magic, but most conveniences come with a price. I've just decided that sometimes the price is too high.
We will all pass someday into the great beyond. Question is...how will we go, what can we do now to make this life and the end of it as healthy and fufilled as possible? I hope plastics and chemicals are never recognized as a *natural* cause of death. I wonder... is that possiblity is really so surprising?

The best thing we can all do is keep trying, stay curious, support and encourage eachother through this funky time we call life.

Write it down

Write down why you want to change your environment, when you are going to change it and how you will go about making the changes. Write down how this makes you feel.

Why:_____
_____
_____
_____

When:_____

How:_____
_____
_____
_____

Feeling:_____
_____
_____
_____
_____
_____

Sign_____

Date_____/_____/_____

Check List
Things to Remove and Replace
Simple goals toward a healthier environment.

- [ ] Toothbrush and floss.
- [ ] Ice cube trays..
- [ ] Kitchen utensils, (Spatuala, Ladel, Strainers, Measuring devices, etc.) Cutting boards.
- [ ] Shopping Bags.
- [ ] Food storage containers, including lunch boxes
- [ ] Toilet paper.
- [ ] Sponges and brushes.
- [ ] Cleaning supplies (Laundry, Dish, and surface cleaners).
- [ ] Clothing (especially under garments).
- [ ] Coated (non-stick) cookware.
- [ ] Deoderants, Lotions, Fragrances and other personal care products.
- [ ] Any plastic drinking container.
- [ ] Baby toys.
- [ ] Candles, Sprays, Plug ins and other Deoderizers.

Add your own

Here's what you'll find after just a few changes:

- Improved mood! It feels good to know what you are allowing in your environment.
- A sense of relief. Now that you know the bad and how to fix it, you'll feel more in charge.
- A sense of purpose. You'll be looking for the next thing to swap. Making it a challenge keeps it fun.
- Sharing. You'll want to share your newfound knowledge and challenge with everyone.
- Healthier. I personally noticed that my environment felt cleaner and I started feeling better.
- Confident. Knowing you are putting in the work and taking the steps to clean up your environment will give you a new sense of confidence in your surroundings.

Everyone's journey is a bit different, but health or lack thereof is something we all experience at one time or another. Getting older has really brought that home for me. Just taking the first step is half the battle. I love cooking more than ever now that most of the toxins are gone from my kitchen. I still hate doing dishes though. Lol.

Remember: Start small. Don't blow it by overwhelming yourself with a giant list attached to a ginormous bill. Ask me how well that goes… I almost didn't start. And, don't listen to the nay sayers who all talk about how, "We are all gonna die someday anyway". It's how I live that matters to me. Besides, we all have a lot to live for and contribute to the next generation.

My parting advice to you is to stay positive and laugh as often as you can. Here are some quotes I reach for when I am getting discouraged or feeling worn down:

"Change what you can, accept what you can't, and have the wisdom to know the difference." — *Unknown*
"Focus on the things you can control and let go of the rest." — *Roy T. Bennett*
"You cannot always control what goes on outside. But you can always control what goes on inside." — *Wayne Dyer*
"Laughter is timeless, imagination has no age, and dreams are forever." — Walt Disney
"Laughter is an instant vacation." — Milton Berle
"Laughter is the shortest distance between two people." — Victor Borge

"A day without laughter is a day wasted." — Charlie Chaplin

"Reach for gratitude. You can always find it where you last left it." K. Savelesky

And with that, I'll be off. I have another thought to think and another book (or 5) to write.

See you on the flip side :)

To those I've never met, but owe so much!

I want to acknowledge the Health Researchers, Clinicians, Doctors and most especially, the Podcasters that give us incredible interviews with these professionals. Thank you for making information so accessible. Without you, thousands of people would continue to suffer in the dark without the light of hope and without a compass for positive change.

Dr. Rhonda Patrick Ph.D

Andrew Huberman M.A. Ph.D

Dr. Paul Saladino M.D. IFMCP

Dr. Josh Axe DNM, DC, CNS

Dr. Peter Osborne PScD, DACBN

Dr. John Campbell Ph.D

Steven Bartlett of "The Diary of a CEO"

Nicolas Verhoeven of Physionic

Mikhaila Peterson

    Marie Claire Haver MD I have the most fabulous doctor because of you!

And finally! Thank you...

Joe Rogan of the "Joe Rogan Experience"

Started us on this journey all those years ago watching your first interview

of Dr. Rhonda Patrick Ph.D.

Who knew :)

About the Author

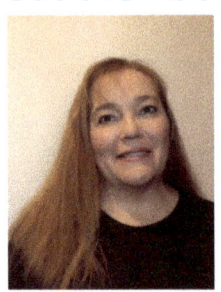

I have been on this awesome planet for 53-years. I have been married to my wonderful husband, supporter and co health adventurer for 30-years. We are parents of 2 amazing adult kids and grandparents of 1 beautiful granddaughter. The constant changes in opinions and science findings on our health drives me bananas. We all have a framework of "normal" and blinders on regarding things that are a fundamental part of our everyday lives. We have been led to believe that "generally recognized as safe" is good enough. Most of us have been deceived, are ignorant and are addicted by the "cheap and easy" life. I'm just as guilty as anyone that reads this book. My goal in writing it is to rip off the blind fold and create a totally doable plan to "end the madness". I encourage you to take back control of your life and health. It's a journey that I hope you will take with me and even have a little fun along the way. Together we can create awareness. Together we can be a positive force for those who need this journey too.

Thank you for sharing your time with me :)

Just finished reading 'Spank The Tomato' and found it really practical. The author does a great job breaking down how to reduce toxins in your home without making it overwhelming. Instead of telling you to throw everything out at once, you get a clear step-by-step plan.

The checklists are actually useful, and I appreciate that the author shares real experiences rather than just theory. It's a quick read that gives you actionable steps you can start using right away.

Perfect for anyone wanting to make healthier choices for their home and family. Straight to the point and genuinely helpful.

-Teigen -Newcastle Wyoming

The book was worth the read and enjoyable.
Michael Byres -Aberdeen Scottland

This book is a quick read jam packed with so much great information. I would recommend it to anyone who is just getting started on their wellness journey and doesn't know where to begin.
-Emily T. -Texas

I found this book extremely interesting, well written, thought provoking and potentially life changing.

I think so many people are oblivious to the harmful products on offer to us and believe if they are sold as 'safe and beneficial' then would never doubt it, I recommend this book to them.

There are so many people questioning how serious health problems are affecting this generation but can not put their finger on how or why, I recommend this book to them.

There are people who want to change so many parts of their lifestyle but find it an impossible task, not even knowing which steps to take first, I recommend this book to them.

Martyn Skillern -United Kingdom

A quick read with lots of great ideas for anyone who is thinking about simple ways to live a healthy life

Chris Hickman, certified arborist -California

Connect with me:

https://discord.gg/gJJXaS3HPq

This book was written utilizing components from Reedsy and revised with help from members of The Next Big Writer

First published by Spank The Tomato LLC 2025
Copyright © 2025 by K. Savelesky

www.ingramcontent.com/pod-product-compliance
Lightning Source LLC
Chambersburg PA
CBHW052131030426
42337CB00028B/5120